The Small Book of Million Dollar Golf Tips

54 of the Most Game Changing Golf Secrets EVERY Golfer Needs to Know but NOBODY Tells You

Jasmin Cull

And

Diana West

How to get the most out of this book

To get the most out of this book, I've included two FREE bonuses.

#1 The Small Book of Million Dollar Golf Tips Video Series ($97 Value)

These are the companion videos to this book. If you're a visual learner, you'll want to watch these videos immediately to speed up how quickly you learn these tips.

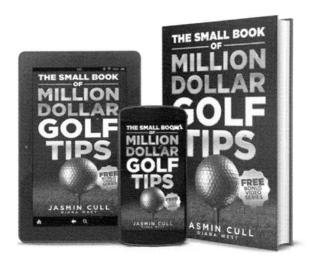

#2 Golf Tips Daily Email ($30 Value)

Follow along as I continue my journey to the PGA tour. Each morning you'll receive a new daily tip or something helpful I've discovered I'd like to share with you. I'll also include stories from the road, and an inside look at what it's like to move up in the golf ranks.

SCAN the QR code below or go to **Jasmincull.com/bonus** to get immediate access to your two free bonuses.

Jasmincull.com/bonus

Table of Contents

Intro: Are you ready to play the best golf of your life?

Golf is a magical game.

In just one week, your entire life can change.

I remember back in 2018 when fellow Canadian Corey Connors won a six man playoff to Monday qualify for a spot on the PGA. One week later he won his first PGA event, pocketed 1.3 million dollars and earned a spot at the Masters.

Then, Sam Burns, 7 strokes behind in the 2022 Charles Schwaab Challenge, ends up in a playoff hole with Scottie Scheffer, and drains a 38 foot putt to win the whole thing.

My favorite reminder, however, of how anything can happen in golf happened last year, when I caddied for one of my friends who was in Canadian Q School qualifying.

Ryan Gerard happened to be in the group.

I didn't think much of it at the time.

His game looked like a lot of other guys I knew.

Fast forward to early 2023.

I get a notification on my phone from the PGA about the four people who Monday qualified for the Honda Classic.

Ryan Gerard happened to be one of them. He ended up making the cut, finishing top 10 and was guaranteed a spot in the next tour event a week later.

At that event, he finished 11th.

Incredible.

That's what I love about golf.

Just one week can make a world of difference.

And in one week, your entire golf game can change too.

That's why I wrote this book.

To show you how just 20 percent of the secrets in golf, what I call **Million Dollar Tips**, can lead to an 80 percent improvement in your game.

Maybe that's breaking 80 this year or winning your first tournament.

Maybe it's healing your back and being so physically strong golf becomes a joy again.

Whatever your goal, reaching it comes down to two critical things, things everyone but the pros get wrong.

Get these two things right and your game will improve so fast, your friends won't recognize you.

People that wouldn't give you the time of day before will suddenly be calling you for tips, asking you to play tournaments, and just wanting to hang out.

It's crazy, but it's true.

How do I know?

Some of you might know my story.

In 2020 at the age of 37, I told my friends and family about my ridiculous dream - to play professional golf on the PGA Tour.

My friends laughed, my mom laughed, pretty much everyone laughed.

Yet, less than 3 years later I was sitting in 5th place day one at the Toronto Player's Tour against golfers with a decade more experience than me.

How could a 37 year old full time former volleyball player and construction worker with three years experience play professional golf?

The answer is I had to get good and I had to get good fast.

What you'll find in this book are the "critical shortcuts", the 20 percent of golf strategy that will give you 80 percent of the results, I learned over the past 3 years.

Like my 1-2, 1-2 rhythm trick.

It's what I used to get my backswing smooth instead of moving before the club came forward.

And the **instant back pain fix** that's been literally lifesaving for me. I've used it more than 100 times over the past year, and each time it's allowed me to keep training, keep competing, and continue to play without pain.

Most of the tricks in this book can be implemented quickly, leading to what feels like a magical improvement in your game.

Others won't feel right at first.

They'll take some trying out to get used to.

I still remember a late night lesson with my swing coach Chris Mcclure this past December.

I had just finished a 10 hour day renovating a home in Toronto. I was beat. But when I put the club in my hand, I was energized.

Everything felt perfect.

I was hitting shot after shot within inches of each other.

I was hitting so consistently Chris yawned and said, "well this is boring."

The next day I showed up for my final lesson of the year with him before heading to Florida.

He made one change to my hand placement and suddenly everything felt like garbage.

Balls were flying everywhere.

"*What the heck*?!" I remember thinking.

I could see how McClure's change could benefit me in the future, but I wasn't ready to force it.

Instead, I incorporated it slowly, trying it some days, not forcing it others.

And that's exactly how I want you to use this book.

Take it out on the course with you. Use your phone to pull up the videos included with this book, and give them a try in real time while you're out playing.

Some of them will work the first time you try them. Others might feel awkward and confusing at first.

Try everything once and keep the things that feel right over time.

But most of all go out there and love every moment of it.

Golf is the most beautiful sport I've ever played with the most generous, most welcoming people.

Get out there, play, and make your next round count.

Jasmin Cull

May 2023

Part 1: What is the one thing in golf EVERY amateur gets wrong?

Do you want to hit more greens?

Do you want to set up your shot perfectly to give you the best chance of par everytime?

Then you have to do the one thing correctly that every amateur golfer gets wrong.

You don't need to swing perfectly, putt perfectly, or play perfectly to shoot par.

There's just one thing you need to do consistently if you want to start out performing everyone else.

What is it?

Tiger said it best.

"I'm not going to out-ball-strike you to death; I'm not going to out-putt you to death; but there's no reason why I can't out-think you," he told Golf Digest.

"Course management over the course of my career has allowed me to win as many tournaments as I have."

It's about out thinking the course.

It's about losing the "go for it mentality" and playing the right club and the right line for the right situation.

"I've always felt I should never make a mental mistake.

We're under no time pressure, no one's trying to rip our heads off—there's no reason I can't go without making a mental mistake the rest of my career," Tiger shared.

If you visualize each hole as you want to play it, you're going to break numbers you never thought possible.

Begin by asking yourself a simple question before each tee.

Secret #1 How do I best take advantage of this hole

What do you think Tiger does when he gets to the hole? He plans from the green back. He asks himself, *"How do I get there? What shot am I going to play in?"* He uses that info to pick what club he's going to hit off the tee and what swing he's going to make.

When you step up to the tee, look at the flag and ask yourself *"How am I going to get there?"*

Then, work backwards.

For example, where do I want to putt from to have the best chance at making it?

What shot do I want to hit to get the ball in that exact position for that putt? Where do I need to drive it from the tee to make that shot possible?

As the great Greg Norman writes:

> *If I know, for instance, that the pin on a par-four hole is cut on the right side of the green, behind a bunker, then the best approach to that pin will usually be from the left side of the fairway, with a shot that will not have to cross over sand.*

Thus, I'll want to hit a tee shot to that left side, assuming there's no dire trouble to dissuade me. This usually means I'll tee my ball at the extreme right side of the teeing area and aim slightly leftward, toward position A.

I recommend that you do this type of 'backward thinking' on any hole where you can see the location of the flagstick from the tee. It's a bit like playing pool - you use the shot at hand to set up the ideal situation for your next shot.

Now if you're shaking your head saying "how the heck am I supposed to know that?

This is the first time I've played this course," I get it.

If you can't see the pin from the tee, there's nothing on Youtube on the course or you're showing up at the last minute to play, you're not going to know much about the holes you're playing.

I've only been playing this game 3 years so most of the courses I play, I'm playing for the first time too.

My first tournament this year was so cold and so wet, they closed the course beforehand so we couldn't even get a practice round.

I had to go in blind, and do the best I could.

AllI I had was a tiny drawing of the course on the back of my scorecard.

For those situations, use the yardage marker to visualize as best you can.

The yardage marker lets you know the exact distance from the marker to the center of the green. From there, you can figure out how to best play the upcoming tee shot until you can see the pin.

For instance, if I know it's a tough hole, say, 400 yards and I know I can carry my driver 330 off the tee, then I can start planning how to play that hole.

I think about what the wind is doing.

Is it on my face or is it behind my back?

What are my strengths today based on warming up at the range before play?

Am I pulling the ball more or am I fading the ball more? What's my miss today?

So if I'm playing that hole and hitting my full distance off the tee I'd have say 60 plus yards left.

That is not good because to hit 60 yards is maybe a ¾ swing for me. I don't want to leave myself with that distance.

It's very finesse and leaves a lot of chances for missing. Instead, I'd hit a 3 wood or shorter iron off the tee so I'd have a comfortable 100 yards or more to hit to the green.

Worse case scenario, you can rehearse these holes in your mind right there at the tee before you play them.

Secret Summary: Work Backwards. Visualize. Asking yourself *How do I best take advantage of this hole?*

Secret #2 Choose your weapons like you aren't as good as you really are

If I asked a group what the biggest mistake their friends make on the course, they'd probably say picking the wrong club and blowing it from the tee.

Why?

It's pretty common for guys like that to believe they are much better than they are. The result? Picking clubs they see the pros using and getting into sticky situations.

Don't be like those guys.

Instead, choose your weapons on the course as if you aren't quite as good as you are.

This is a simple **way to cut as much as 5 strokes from your next round**, because you will play the safe club and ensure far more pars.

I have a series on my Instagram called "What Club Wednesday." It's where I talk with my followers about what club they are using to hit certain shots.

The biggest mistake I see over and over is golfers choosing clubs like they are a professional.

What ends up happening is they choose a driver instead of an iron they can lay up with and hit a hazard they would have been safe from.

Here's what I mean.

Today I was looking at a 400 yard par 4, wind directly in my face at 30 mph.

At the 130 yard mark the fairway narrows and there's a hazard to the right and to the left.

The smart shot would be a low 2 iron right up the middle. I'd avoid the hazards and have a safe 150 to 170 to the hole.

Then I'd have a decent birdie chance.

Instead, I decided to hit a driver and ended up triple bogeying the hole.

Ouch.

The decision off the tee costs me 3 shots instead of no shots.

Simple course management would have allowed me to play that hole much, much better.

Secret Summary: Play it safe and you'll end up outperforming everyone. Choose clubs as though you're not quite as good as you really are.

Secret #3 How to break 80 in your spare time without going to the range or picking up a single club

The biggest question I get asked is how I was able to get good so fast, while playing so little.

I haven't told a lot of people how I really did it because most people won't like my answer. I think most people want to hear that I have some secret talent that allowed me to go pro in just two years.

The thing is, when I started training to play golf professionally, my days were like everyone else's.

I woke up early and went to work until late.

I had weekends and nights available to train and play.

So how?

I used technology, and not in the way you might think.

It wasn't something special from my equipment.

I was playing with clubs I bought for $100 over at Sports Chek.

And it wasn't something crazy I learned at lessons.

I could only play or take lessons when I could afford it, which was nowhere near how much I really wanted to play.

What I did can be copied by anyone who has a phone and knows the difference between a good and bad golf swing.

I perfected my game through videos I made and watched on my phone.

I've broken it down for you into four steps:

1. I hired a swing coach
2. I videoed everytime I trained or played
3. I watched my videos over and over again, mentally rehearsing how I wanted my swing to look, where I wanted the ball to go, and how I wanted to feel during each part of my play.
4. I copied people who were better than me

Steps 1 through 3 are pretty self explanatory. Step 4 is where the real fun is. Because for those that can't afford lessons yet or just don't have the time, step 4 can help you get a pretty incredible swing.

I break it down more in Secret #4.

Secret Summary: Film yourself every time you practice so you can actually see what you are doing and compare it to what you want to do.

Secret #4 How to perfect your swing without lessons, practice at the range, or taking any swings at all

When you watch a video and then visualize yourself performing what you saw, your body learns as though you were there at the range practicing.

It has to do with the way our brain works.

Did you know...

When we practice something in our minds, it is very similar to if we physically did the task ourselves?

It's true and verified by numerous studies.

Take for example a study done by Dr. Blaslotto at the University of Chicago in 1996 on visualization.

Randomly selected students were split into three groups.

Group #1 was told not to touch a basketball for 30 days.

Group #2 was told to shoot free throws for half an hour a day for 30 days.

Group #3 was told to come to the gym everyday and spend half an hour with their eyes closed visualizing themselves making free throws.

The researchers couldn't believe the results.

Group #1 made no improvement.

Nothing surprising there.

Group #2 made a 24% improvement (not bad at all for 30 minutes of sweating).

Group #3 made a 23% improvement.

No sweating. No gear required. No frustrations of practice. Just visualizing.

This is incredible news because it means you can get better just by thinking about getting better.

It's also at the heart and soul of the 80/20 Pareto Principle - 20% of your effort leads to 80% of your results.

What does this have to do with golf?

You're going to mimic this study by mentally picturing yourself going through the motions used by other golfers.

Ten time PGA tour winner Justin Rose said "It's strange to think you are training your brain to relax, evolve, and build confidence."

But that's exactly what you're doing.

Training yourself to feel and move like a pro by watching how they play over and over.

The basics are pretty simple.

1. Watch videos of golfers you want to golf like.
2. Video your swing
3. Compare your swing to the gofers you want to swing like, and finally
4. Continue practicing the swing mentally and physically until it feels right

You never even have to step foot on the golf course to do this. You can practice this anywhere, and you don't even need to have a club all of the time.

You're just looking at the motion and seeing how it compares to the swing of great golfers.

Can you see how these "Mind Movies" as I call them can make a huge difference in your golf game?

Secret Summary: Mental training can be nearly equal to physical training without the strain, the expense, or the frustration that comes from being on the course. The investment is small but the payoff can be huge.

Secret #5 Why every smart golfer needs their own collection of mind movies

Beyond not needing to spend money, drive anywhere, or have equipment to do mental review, this kind of practice is especially easy on the body and one of the ways you can stay sharp even when you're injured.

That's why every smart golfer needs to create their own personal video library or "Mind Movies" as I call them.

Find a few good videos of every skill you're seeking to improve. Include a few good swings you'd like to copy from several different golfers like Tiger Woods in his heyday, Rory Mcllroy, Adam Scott, and Nelly Korda.

And you'll want to include videos from all different trouble spots out on the course.

If you're struggling to find good videos, message me on Instagram @JasminCullGolf.

I'll point you in the right direction.

Secret Summary: Create your own library of Mind Movies to refer back to daily.

Secret #6 A simple rhythm trick to swing smooth on every shot

"Golf is a game best played in the subconscious." – Alister MacKenzie, designer of Augusta and Cypress Point

A study of 75 PGA professionals found they have no swing thoughts at all.

Instead, if they did think of something, it was to focus on a spot a few inches in front of the ball to encourage swinging through.

To get to that point however, they spent hundreds of hours practicing their swing.

If you don't have hundreds of hours to practice, but need to get your swing into your subconscious faster, there's a trick.

Have you ever found yourself hearing a song and being instantly transported to a memory you had hearing that song?

Often you can remember everything about that moment. Where you were, who you were with, and what you were doing.

Music has a powerful effect on recall in your subconscious. It can be an incredible tool for you when golfing.

One of the easiest ways to cement your swing into your subconscious during practice is to put your song to a rhythm like humming a tune or giving yourself a beat.

This has helped me get my backswing down. When I was struggling to take the club back far enough, I put the motion to the rhythm of **1-2, 1-2**.

You can implement it by thinking of a beat or a song at the start of your swing - something smooth that can get you in a rhythm while you're practicing.

When you're out on the course, use that same beat or song to get you right into the same swing pattern.

Secret Summary: Use a beat to cement the rhythm of your swing into your subconscious.

Secret #7 The "No Lesson Needed" self assessment trick to diagnose your swing no matter how crazy it's acting on the course

Ever felt like you've lost your swing?

Ever had those days, weeks or even months when you keep slicing, topping, or hooking the ball and you can't for the life of you figure out why?

If you memorize these self-assessment secrets, you won't waste weeks and months wondering what's going wrong with your swing.

You can figure it out instantly, just by watching the flight of your ball.

It doesn't matter how wild or crazy your swing is, you just need to know what's happening at impact to solve all of your problems including curing your top, your slice or your hook.

Everything you need to know is in the flight path of the ball. Once you see what's happening with your ball flight, you can work backwards from there.

The best video I've ever seen on self diagnosing swings was done by Danny Maude. If you haven't seen his Youtube yet, check him out. He's an incredible instructor with a knack for breaking things down simply.

No matter what shot you're playing whether you're dribbling it along the ground, topping it, slicing to the right, hooking to the left, you can know exactly what is going wrong if you understand what is happening the moment the ball hits the club face.

If you're hitting the ball well, striking it square at a perfect 90 degrees to target, your ball will fly straight.

If you're not hitting it straight and are in the slice or hook family, it can only be one of a few problems. And if you diagnose those, you have a magical recipe to fix all of your swing problems.

Ball Goes Straight But to the Right

If your ball is going straight to the right - you're hitting the ball too soon and your club is straight to the target at the right.

Ball Curves to the Right

If you're hitting it to the right but it's curving too - you're hitting the ball early again but this time your club face isn't square to the right, it's open. This is what's making your ball go right and then continue to curve right.

Hooking It - Ball Starts Low Then Curves Left

If you're hooking it where the ball starts out low and right and then curves left, again, you're hitting it early but this time the club face is closed.

Ball Flies Straight Left

Ball flies straight to the left, you're catching it late and the club face is completely square to the path.

Ball Pull Hooks - Flies Straight but Curves Left

Ball pull hooks - flies straight but curves left- you're still hitting late and the clubface is closed.

It's a Slice

If you sliced it you're catching the ball late and this time your clubface is open at the end causing the curve.

Thinning the Ball

If you're thinning the ball, you're too shallow and catching it on the way up.

Ball Flight is Super High

If your ball travels super high, you're hitting too steep, catching it slightly on the way up.

Catching the Ground Behind the Golf Ball, Leaving a Shallow Divot

If you catch the ground behind the golf ball but the divot isn't deep, you're hitting it too shallow.

Ball Traveling too Low

If the ball travels low, you're coming in too steep

Topping the Ball

If you top the ball, you're also coming too steep

Catching the Ground, Leaving Large Divot

If you hit the ground and the divot is big, again you're coming too steep on your swing.

If you can use these 12 identifiers to diagnose your swing, you will make drastic leaps in your game.

Not only that, but imagine the difference you can make in the way your friends play.

Let's say you have a friend named Mike and they feel like they have lost their golf swing.

They continue to hit the ball to the right and it continues to curve right. What could you tell them to instantly diagnose their swing?

"Hey Mike, you haven't lost your swing, you're hitting it early and your clubface is open."

Now Mike has a very simple solution. Try hitting more to the right.

Now Mike can set up to the ball differently, working on hitting more right. He could make tiny little adjustments until he began hitting perfectly down the fairway.

If one of your friends misses a shot or two, there's nothing really to diagnose.

But, if they are consistently hitting the same way over and over again, turn to these 12 identifiers to help them out.

Secret Summary: You too can be a coach with these 12 identifiers. Give it a shot.

Secret #8 Improve 100% faster than everyone else by using "Random Practice"

If you've been to the range recently you probably went through the typical practice lineup. You might have hit a 7 iron over and over or a 3 wood or driver until it felt good before moving onto the next club.

That's how most people practice actually and there's a better way.

It's called Random Practice, and when baseball professionals tried it, they ended up hitting 57% more pitches than when they first started, double what the other players normally hit.

When we practice with one club over and over, our brain gets used to the repetition and becomes less and less responsive to it. Basically, our brain notices we are doing the same thing over and over and gets bored.

What it really needs is change. That's where Random Practice comes in.

Instead of hitting one club for a while, you're going to mix it up by hitting several other clubs in between the clubs you're practicing on. If you're practicing your driver, you swing with your driver then move onto a wedge, then maybe an iron before going back to your driver.

What this does is force your brain to go back and remember what you are about to do. It has to refocus each time you switch between clubs.

And that's great news! Because the more active your mind is, the faster you learn and the more the information stays with you.

Secret Summary: Use Random Practice at the range. Take several clubs. Switch between them often. Force your mind to stay active and focused. Do this and you can double the effectiveness of your practice session.

Secret #9 Break 90 and lower your scores without changing your grip, hitting the ball further, or messing with your rotation

I once overheard a golfer say the best way to break 90, or even 85, is to play just 14 holes.

Pretty funny.

I'd say the next best way is to prevent double and triple bogeys.

How?

Most double or triple bogeys start because a golfer makes a single bad shot. To make up for it, they take a hero shot.

That's when more bad things happen.

Instead of playing a safe shot they instead go for a shot that would need a miracle to make it.

What was just one bad shot and either a bogey or a par turns into a double or triple bogey.

For example, let's say you've made a bad shot and the fairway is just 50 yards away.

Normally you'd use a sand wedge and it would be an easy little punchout. But in this situation you have trees hanging over the fairway.

The safe shot would be to try a seven or an eight iron here for a nice low shot that runs out of the rough and onto the fairway.

Secret Summary: When you make one bad shot, accept it. Don't be a hero. Play a safe shot immediately after. Start the next hole fresh.

Secret #10 Same with bunkers

Hit the bunker? No big deal. Accept it and play the safe shot immediately after. Take a look at where you are at. Where is the fairway? Where is the green? What is the easiest, safest shot you can take to get back on track? That's the one to take.

Let's say we're in a greenside bunker.

Once you've planned your shot, now it's time for the set up.

The biggest mistake people make is not feeling out the bunker. When you get in the bunker and stand over the shot, wiggle your feet in the sand.

Does the sand feel shallow or deep?

In shallow sand you keep the face normal so the edge can dig through the sand.

In deep sand, we have to open the club face so the club can bounce through the sand.

Nice bunkers are going to be deep. A lot of golfers will underestimate the loft needed to get out of there.

They keep their club face square or closed. That's a no go here.

Instead we are going to set up and open our club more to the right to give more loft and elevation.

Another benefit of getting more loft is you'll get more bounce with the ball when it lands and really take advantage of the course.

Next you need to feel the weight in your front foot. This is completely different from your normal swing.

When you're ready, swing through!

Let's set it up.

Open your club face. Weight forward on the front foot. Visualize a line in the sand a couple inches behind your ball.

Be confident. Swing with speed.

Secret Summary: Tell your friends "Bring some sunscreen cause you're never getting off the beach!" Then, when you're in the bunker take the safe shot. Assess the sand, get your weight in your front foot, and swing with speed.

Secret #11 What about a fairway bunker?

The fairway bunker you're going to need more distance and less loft. How are we going to do that?

First, take more club.

The ball is not going to travel as far as you think it will.

Once you're stable in the sand, unlike the greenside bunker, take your regular swing catching the ball first and the sand second or the ball will go nowhere.

Secret summary: Use extra club and swing like any other shot

Secret #12 How to eliminate three putts for good even if your grip is wrong, your swing is out of whack, and you haven't been playing well

This secret is about mastering the long putt.

That way, even if you make a bad first shot, if you master the long putt, you can still save par.

Just having this in your wheelhouse makes you feel more confident so you make better, safer shots on the course.

The secret here is not to spend too much time worrying about the slope. Yes, up and down will affect the ball.

What's more important is to focus on the speed of the ball.

Let go of figuring out the complexity of the break for now. If it's breaking left to right, pick a point three or four feet left of the flag and the goal is to get it there.

Take a few good practice strokes. Visualize the speed of the ball moving towards the hole.

Does the length of the stroke feel like it's going to get you to the hole?

Once you've done the planning, you have a rough estimate of how hard you're going to hit it to get it close, now comes the crucial part - striking it near the middle.

Strike the ball somewhere else and it's going to drop off and fall short of where you need it to go.

To do it, find a point on the back of the ball. I'm talking about a really small point, almost like a dimple back there.

Hit that dimple with the center of the putter face.

Secret Summary: Master the long putt to avoid future 3 putts. It's all about getting the right speed in the long putt. Pick a spot three or four feet to the hole and get the ball there.

Secret #13 Don't get fooled by the sucker pin

Look at how a hole is designed.

A lot of holes give you the option to cut the corner to shorten the hole. The pin can look juicy but really it's attempting to fool you into a really bad shot.

I call these sucker pins.

They make you think you can outsmart the course.

Don't fall for it.

Aim for the safe zone, where the most amount of green is.

Go for the safest section and put it on the dance floor.

Secret Summary: If it looks too good to be true, it probably is. Keep it simple golfer.

Secret #14 How to make par when you're in between distances

When you're out on the golf course and you're trying to put a score together, sometimes you'll find yourself between distances.

For example, maybe you're 155 yards from the flag.

That's either a massive 9 iron or a soft 8 iron.

I'm guilty of trying to take the shorter club and smash it to the pin. But the problem with that is trying to swing harder changes up your swing and could lead to miss hitting the ball.

The solution is to go with an extra club and grip down on it to take a little speed off the swing.

You're still going to pick your line. You're still going to know what shot you're going to hit. And you're still going to be fully confident when you're standing over the ball.

The only change is in the club selection and where you grip it to take a little speed off it.

Of course, if there's trouble behind the green and a chance of hitting it through the back you're not going to do this.

It's not such a safe shot anymore if that's the case.

The majority of the time when you're stuck between distances, go with an extra club, grip down on it a couple inches, and commit.

Secret Summary: Don't get married to one club if you're stuck between distances. Club up and swing smoothly.

Secret #15 Have 3 swings for every wedge

Most golfers use just one swing for their wedges.

That leaves them with some hard to make shots on partial distances.

Changing the distance of your shot can be as simple as having 3 different swings - a 50%, 75%, and full, 100% swing.

1. Half Swing - bring your arm parallel to the ground, or a 9 o'clock position. Swing through half the clock over to the 3 o'clock position or right at your hips.
2. Three quarter swing - This will get you an extra 10 yards or so. Bring your arm back to 11 then swing to 1 or around chest level.
3. Full swing. Take it all the way back and follow all the way through, ending up at your shoulder.

Practice in an empty field or at the driving range to see what distances you get with each swing.

This will give you options around the green and make you much more lethal out there.

Secret Summary: Have more weapons for each distance you're trying to hit.

Secret #16 Hit more greens and fairways in regulation with the "2-Foot Aiming Rule"

Being closer to the green means hitting closer to the hole.

In order to do it, you have to overcome one of the most common (yet simply fixed) errors in golf.

I'm talking about how you aim.

I once heard a story about a pro golfer who participated in a lot of Pro/Am events.

That's where 1 pro is paired with three or four amateurs.

In every single one of those rounds, they noticed someone misaligned at the tee.

Sometimes it was the pro.

The reason?

They were aiming their feet at the target.

But what good is that going to do? If you aim your feet at the target, where is the clubface aligned?

To the right!

Instead, get your feet aligned a little to the left of the target line, parallel to it.

To make it a habit, you're going to perform the same aiming strategy as part of your pre-shot routine.

Take a look at how Jack Nicholaus does it:

Step 1: He looks at the target from behind the ball.

Step 2: He picks a spot a few feet ahead of his ball in line with that target. That's his first target.

Step 3: He walks to the ball and sets the club face behind it so he's aiming at the first target, the intermediate point.

Aligning the club with something 2 feet away is much easier than aiming 30 yards away.

Secret Summary: Always have a close target just in front of you. That will keep you from aiming your feet at the target.

Secret #17 How to stop hitting the ground before the ball and strike your irons better than ever before (easy fix)

Hitting the ground before the ball is one of the most frustrating shots in golf.

It's a weak shot. It's inconsistent.

The problem comes from shifting too much weight during your backswing.

When that happens, you end up striking the ground first before the ball.

Take heart.

There's an easy fix.

When you use it, you'll be amazed at what one small change in form can do for your game.

You'll gain more distance and strike the ball pure everytime.

It starts with ball position. Record yourself or ask a friend to watch how you're lining up.

Is it in the right position for the right club?

High loft clubs like your wedges and 9 iron you'll line the ball up dead center of your sternum.

Mid irons you'll line up about 1 ball to the left of your sternum.

Long irons you'll line up about 1 ½ balls to the left of your sternum.

You don't want to go further than that with your irons or you'll end up hitting high.

Once you've lined up correctly, you're going to stay fixed to that line, rotating around the center column of your swing. This prevents the weight shift responsible for striking the ground early.

Then in the downswing, you're going to uncoil your weight to the left as you rotate your body. Viola. Use these tips and you'll be much, much happier with your strike.

You're going to hit your irons better than before, hitting farther than before and with more consistency. You'll avoid heavy shots, fat shots, and other horrendous moves no one wants in their game.

Secret Summary: Get in the right position for the right club.

Secret #18 How to never miss a short putt again

Legendary golfer Bobby Jones once said that when it comes down to one shot, nothing is more frightening than having to make a short putt.

Because the putt is so short, there's this expectation that we SHOULD make it.

So we put tremendous pressure on ourselves, tense up, and end up missing it.

The secret to killing tension and putting fluid and free is to keep your fine motor muscles and eyes continually moving.

Have you noticed how Ricky Fowler hovers over his putter until he hits it at the last minute?

Before every single one of Fowler's putts, right before the moment he pulls the trigger, Fowler lifts the putterhead a fraction of an inch off the ground.

By lifting the putter, he's releasing the tension, and increasing his chances of a nice, smooth putting stroke.

Jordan Spieth has a little forward press that keeps his motion going.

He rocks the handle just slightly toward the target when he starts his stroke.

You can wiggle your toes, tap your putter or copy Fowler and Spieth.

Most importantly, just before you start your stroke, exhale, let the tension out and sink that putt.

Secret Summary: Release nerves by moving, starting the stroke, and exhaling as you nail that putt.

Secret #19 How to make even your worst chip shots end up closer to the pin

I've heard a lot from frustrated golfers whose handicap is decently low but they feel like they lose at least six shots a round from chipping.

So I'm going to show you a simple way to make your chipping good enough even your worst chip shots end up closer to the pin.

This technique makes the path of your club closer to straight back and straight through.

There's also less rotation on the swing, giving you more control.

What you are going to do is stand closer and raise the handle of your club so it's more vertical.

Why?

The farther you hit away from the ball, the path of the club is more inwards.

The club face also rotates open and closed more. This is much harder to control.

Stand in much closer, raise the handle up and even when you do have a duff shot it will end up much, much better.

Pretty simple right?

Secret Summary: By lifting up on the shaft, we get the heel of the club out of the equation. Meaning? Better control and better results.

Secret #20 The Tiger Woods "Master's Method" to making the best putts of your life

A lot of amateur golfers want to look at the pin and let their natural athletic ability take over, but a lot of the time, they end up hitting it too far and blowing the hole.

The secret to becoming a great golfer is to focus not on the pin, but on where you want the ball to land.

I like how Steve Williams describes it, talking about Tiger's 2015 "Greatest chip in Masters history."

"Once we got to the ball, I was very relieved to see Tiger had a shot and could get it on the green and most likely make a 4. Tiger had a long look at the shot and pointed out an old pitch mark on the green and asked me what I thought if he landed it in that area. Incredibly, when he pitched the shot it landed exactly on the pitch mark. When the ball started rolling towards the hole I thought, 'You know what? We can escape with a 3 here.' What happened next incredible. I was so pumped I went to high-five Tiger and we missed.

The key to making more shots is to get the ball where you planned.

Start by focusing on the spot you want the ball to land.

If you're playing a popular course you've seen played on TV you can take this technique to the next level.

You can copy top golfers who have birdied the same hole you are playing. Look at the spot they aimed for and how they played the hole to birdie.

See if you can follow the same path.

Secret Summary: Take your focus off the pin. Focus instead on where you want the ball to land and the rest is history.

Secret #21 The only phrase you need to remember to get out of the bunker and up and down more often

Why are bunker shots so hard?

Because we make them that way.

Hundreds of thoughts flowing through your mind before taking a shot will make anyone underperform.

Instead, one simple phrase could help you hit much more solid bunker shots and get up and down more often.

It's really, really simple and you can do it next time you play.

Get the sand on the green.

How it works is when you stand over the golf ball, forget about the ball.

Instead, focus on taking the sand around the ball and putting it on the green.

The two things this does is help with the approach angle you're taking on the ball. It keeps you from hitting too steep and into the sand so you instead hit through the sand .

Second, it gives you a good idea of how much speed you need.

If you're the type of golfer who is noncommittal and a decelerator in the bunkers, you'll often come up short.

Getting the sand on the green helps you commit and helps you focus on moving through your follow through position and getting the right speed in the impact area.

Try this next time you're out to hit more solid bunker shots and get up and down more often.

Secret Summary: Get the sand on the green

Secret #22 The "5 Min-Fix" to stop shanking

Everyone freaks out about shanking.

Shanking strikes when you least expect it and there's no explanation why.

One minute you'll be playing well, the next, you can't hit a ball right to save your life.

But shanking can be so easy to fix if you see what's happening.

You don't need to hit a thousand balls or take lessons from many different pros.

This "5 Min Fix" is all you need.

Even if right now you don't shank, remember this because when it happens, if you don't know what to do, weeks could go by and that can completely ruin your game and your confidence.

Shanking happens when the ball hits the hosel of your golf club.

That's the part where the shaft connects to the club.

If you hit it, the ball doesn't fly very high and squirts off to the right. The worst part about the shank though is it feels like you've made a good shot.

The ball just isn't ending up in the direction you want it.

But if you look at your club, you'll see little marks on the hosel where the ball has been hitting.

A lot of beginners who shank think they are leaving the club face open. But that's not it.

Look for ball marks on the hosel to see if you are shanking.

Now think about what club you're shanking with?

Are you doing it with a driver? There's no hosel on a driver so that's probably not happening.

What about a 4 iron?

Not that one either?

So what have you been shanking with?

Most likely the shorter clubs.

The shorter the club is, the more you have to bend over to use it. When you do that, your mass is hanging over your toe line.

If you start with the weight in the middle of your feet, when you bend over, now the weight goes to your toes.

That means I'm closer to the ball now and what happens when I swing? I shank it.

Basically, when your body gets ahead of your toe line, that's one of the main reasons for shanking.

You might be using a little more arm too, since shanking happens with the shorter clubs.

It takes just three steps to fix the shank.

Step 1: Stand taller. Maybe you're shanking with an 8 iron down. It's happening with the shorter clubs because you're leaning over too far. So stand taller. Think about it. If you feel your weight in your toes as you hit, you're probably leaning over too far. Use a little knee bend to get your motion more up and down instead of bending over to the ground.

Step 2: Center your weight in your feet. Feel your weight evenly across each foot. Not in your toes or in the balls of your feet, but spread evenly throughout your foot.

Step 3: Hit the ball by thinking "back heel", "forward heel" as you swing. What's happening is you're rotating from one heel to the the next as you swing.

There's no need to worry about the dreaded shanks.

If you can stand tall with shorter clubs, you will probably never shank another ball in your life.

Secret Summary: Stand tall, center your weight, think "back heel", "forward heel" as you swing. This is your official shanks cure.

Secret #23 How to trick yourself out of the yips with a single question

Do you remember when Ernie Els three putted from six feet on one hole and then missed a series of mind bogglingly easy short putts on others?

Yikes.

He got the yips.

As Ernie described, there was some sort of short circuit going on in his brain. Where he can putt fine practicing, but he gets on the course and suddenly for no reason, he can't play.

That's the Yips in a nutshell.

Your brain and your muscles get scrambled. Once your muscles start running the wrong program it's like a scratch on a record. Over time, that scratch gets deeper and deeper.

The cure lies in your ability to change where you give your attention.

A lot of golfers get stuck by putting a lot of attention on themselves.

They think *Is my grip right? How are my shoulders and wrist moving?* These are all technical thoughts.

The more technical you get the more you reduce your ability to visualize where the ball will go.

You become stuck in the left brain instead of the more creative right brain.

This is a sure fire way to get a good case of the yips.

If you spend all your time training your attention to focus on technique, guess what you will be thinking about on the course?

Technique.

Then you go to the golf course and it doesn't work!

Ugh oh. You go back to the range and try again. It's a vicious cycle.

You can do the opposite.

Train your attention on the golf ball.

The more your attention is on what you want the golf ball to do, the more your body will naturally organize your movements to get it there.

You become looser, more automatic.

You can change your attention by asking the right questions.

Like Tony Robbins says, the quality of your questions dictates the quality of your life.

Instead of asking yourself why am I struggling, why am I slicing, or why am I not hitting the green (all training you to think about technique), let's flip the script.

Try this sentence instead:

What do I need to do to get the ball to my target?

Or what do I need to do to get the ball in the hole?

Asking these visualizing centered questions flips your attention away from technique and into a more creative right brain process.

Try this immediately to protect yourself from or banish a case of the yips you might be struggling with right now!

Secret Summary: Don't be Ernie! Get your attention off technique and onto the ball.

Secret #24 New grip cures the yips (for putting ONLY)

This won't work with your long game, but for putting it's perfect. It's from performance coach Karl Morris.

If you have the Yips while you're putting, you can get out of them immediately by changing your putting grip.

That's because you'll be interrupting the "YIPS" path you've recently created.

By trying something new, you'll completely turn off the misfiring in your muscles that's causing a meltdown in your game.

Skip this for your long game, however.

Your long game is pretty set.

You can't be switching things up randomly, but with putting, there's a million ways to do it.

Here are five different grips you can try:

1. Cross Hand
2. Split Hand
3. The Claw
4. Palm to Palm

5. Arm to Arm

Secret Summary: Next time you get the yips putting, switch your grip and get right back on track.

Secret #25 Pre-shot to stay hot: The Jason Day method to nailing every hole

It's no coincidence the greatest players of all time have an air tight mental game and air tight pre-shot routine. They visualize themselves winning the hole from tee to green on every single shot.

Having the same routine at each hole keeps you focused and on target no matter how many holes you've played.

Tiger Woods has been visualizing since his pre teen years.

Jack Nickalaus has been quoted saying he never hit a shot until he visualized himself nailing it, but probably the example I love most is Jason Day visualizing himself to his first major title at the 2015 PGA Championship.

He would stand behind the ball, close his eyes, and picture his shot in great detail, visualizing the entire flight of it prior to getting into his stance.

The more detailed, the better.

Here's four steps to copy his routine.

1. Get behind the ball and visualize making your shot

For example, start by looking at your ball.

Imagine it soaring through the air, flying all the way to your target. Picture the flight of the ball, how it curves in the air, and bounces and rolls as it lands.

2. Pick a small, intermediate target directly in line with your target but six inches to two feet in front of the golf ball
3. Walk in with your body open relative to the target
4. Square the clubface
5. Take your stance
6. Let the body do what the body knows how to do

Secret Summary: Your body is a machine. If you keep the programming the same, you'll play the same. Master this pre-shot routine to stay hot on every shot.

Secret #26 How to stop mentally blowing games when the pressure is on

When we are playing for money, our adrenalin rises. Our heart rate increases. We play differently.

If you want to play your best, you need to slow it down and get back to normal.

How? By using priming.

It's the idea that one thing can trigger another. It's why visualization works.

Dr. Bob Rotella, Sports Psychologist and one of the top 25 golf instructors of all time as voted by Links Magazine had some great advice for playing under pressure.

Just imagining things you are grateful for can trigger a good mood or get you to calm down in a tough situation.

I like to call it **"Sending yourself on vacation between shots."**

What's unique about golf is we have these long periods of reset in between shots.

Take advantage of them!

After each shot, train your mind to be in a happy mood by imagining walking through your favorite beach as you walk.

Looking at the trees in between shots can do the same thing – it's proven that we are calmer and walk slower in nature compared to urban areas.

The point here is to find a trigger that can instantly calm you down when you find your heart racing. The calmer you are, the better you will play.

Secret Summary: Use the time between shots to "go on vacation" and take a reset.

Part 2: Eliminate back pain

and create a bulletproof body

Secret #27 The lifesaving "full swing cheat" for older golfers and anyone with limited low back mobility

I learned this trick from PT and TPI medical expert Adam Halseth in the video he did with Golf Science lab.

If you're having limited motion in the hip and mid-back, pressure will go instead to your low back.

But that isn't the way our vertebrae are designed.

If you're limited in hip movement, when you go to take your backswing you're gonna keep turning but you'll end up using your lower back to compensate and that's when we get problems.

That's one of the reasons we see so many back injuries on the course.

If you do have limited motion in your swing, here's a quick cheat to get your full swing back without putting pressure on your lower back.

Get lined up and right before you start your backswing, flare your back toe out 20 degrees.

This improves your amount of rotation you have because you are opening up your hip.

Now you can turn your hip over a lot more without using your back to compensate.

Secret Summary: Flare your back toe out 20 degrees to open your stance and get that full swing going again.

Secret #28 Get instant back pain relief even if your pain is so bad you can barely walk

If you've ever been on the course and had pain that shoots down your back, into your butt and legs, there's something you can do about it.

Not only am I going to show you an instant fix for when you throw your lower back out, I'll show you a strategy to make sure it never happens again.

The fix for this is pretty easy to do and most importantly quick.

If you do it right you're going to feel relief right away.

I can't take all the credit for this one.

Diana, who helped me write this book, learned this trick after watching a video from former New York Mets Head Physical Therapist and Assistant Strength coach Jeff Cavaliere.

It has been lifesaving for me.

I can't imagine how much further I would be in my golf career if I had known about this fix and my "Bullet Proof Back Warm-up" back in 2021.

That was when I played my first pro event, and had to take the summer off after throwing my back out on a swing.

I've used it hundreds of times since then to stop even the slightest back flare up.

The relief is instant and I've never missed a tournament since.

This won't work for everyone, but if you have pain like mine and a lot of other golfers this could make a world of difference.

I nicknamed the underlying technique "golfers kickbacks" because it's a move every golfer needs to know.

Here's how to implement them for back pain:

First, lean forward and rub your hands across the low back, you should be able to feel two spots where the bones are prominent.

If you run your fingers just to the outside - and you get all the increase in pain, and tension - then this trick should instantly rid you of your back pain.

Here's how to relieve it:

Get down on the ground and lie on your side.

Then put your hand on your side to stabilize while putting your thumb right on that spot.

From here, all you're going to do is push down with pressure from your thumb, and then move your leg in a certain direction.

If you've been using one, make sure you stop using a lacrosse ball on your back if it's in pain.

You're already inflamed. The lacrosse ball puts too much pressure on the area that's likely to resist what you're trying to do and not help fix it.

Instead you want to use your thumb on the painful spot and top down pressure you can control.

So once your thumb is on that spot, you're going to move your leg forward and bend it until your knee touches the ground.

Once it touches the ground, bring it back to the start point as you straighten it out. Then move it back behind you, into extension.

It's key you get your leg behind the midline of your body and then when you do, you're going to keep your leg straight and lift it towards the ceiling.

Your toes should be pointing a little bit down toward the ground when you do.

Repeat this full motion about 10 times.

What we're doing here is trying to fatigue out the muscle spasm, the trigger point causing back pain.

See if you can burn it out.

You hold that spot one more time, get right back into the position.

Leg is getting back into extension, toes pointed down, abduct it, and hold it, and squeeze as hard as you can.

This back pain could be coming from bad posture or a muscle imbalance, but if you notice you have frequent low back pain, the muscle is probably really, really dang weak.

So this exercise alone might feel like agony.

And you might have trouble doing this exercise or holding your leg up, even if you can squat hundreds of pounds.

When you're done, you should notice immediate relief in the amount of discomfort you feel in that spot.

That gets rid of pain in the short term.

So what to do in the long run?

Secret #29 is the solution.

Secret Summary: Skip the lacrosse ball. Put your thumb on the painful spot in your back and burn it out with abduction kickbacks.

Secret #29 Steal my bulletproof back warm-up routine

My co-author, Diana, is also a former professional athlete and an accomplished powerlifter.

She introduced me to the work of Doctor of Physical Therapy and Squat University founder Dr. Aaron Horschig.

She traveled to his clinic in St. Louis for back pain she had when lifting.

He told her that the traditional way the fitness and rehab world tries to strengthen core and fix back pain is completely backwards.

That's because what most people don't understand is that many people who develop back pain already have strong backs.

What they are lacking is core and spine stability. And doing more back extensions, situps, twists, ab exercises and using the glute ham machine will do little to increase core stiffness.

To protect and stabilize your back you need core stiffness. To get this, you have to train your core differently.

How?

Using the **McGill Big 3.**

The system was invented by Dr. Stuart McGill of Waterloo University.

Over the past few decades he has written extensively on the topic of back injuries and the concept of core stability.

Think of the spine as a flexible rod that needs to be stiffened to bear load. This is the role of the muscles.

When muscles contract they create force and stiffness. It is the stiffness part that is important for stability.

Through his research, McGill has measured athletes who fail to obtain appropriate muscular stiffness around the spine by coordinating muscle activation, and their subsequent injuries and pain.

In his years of studying the spine, Dr. McGill has found there to be three specific exercises that most efficiently address all of these areas without placing excessive stresses on the parts of the back that may be aggravated or irritated due to injury. This group of exercises has famously become known as 'The Big 3.'

- Curl-Up

- Side Plank
- Bird-Dog

Get mobile first

If you have tightness in the hips and thoracic spine, it can limit your movement during exercise. What happens then?

Your back takes over.

Not good!

Use the Cat-Camel exercise before the Big 3 to reduce stiffness and increase mobility of the spine.

Secret Summary: Follow my Bulletproof Back warm-up to strengthen your core and protect your back

- Cat cow - 3 sets of 10 with 20 - 30 seconds rest between each.
- McGill Big 3 - Do 3 sets using a descending pyramid for reps. For example five reps, then three, and finally one to end (each with an 8-10 second hold).
- Rest between each set for 20-30 seconds

Secret #30 How to end back pain for good

If you're doing your Bulletproof Back warm up, you're on your way to correcting back imbalances.

Now it's time to add strength in the right places.

Start by adding 5 minutes of these easy back strengthening exercises.

Do these 3 or 5 times a week if you can, and work your way up to 7 if you're up for the challenge.

What you'll find is within six weeks, you'll be surprisingly strong at any of these.

There are three exercises in total, all done with bodyweight for now.

1. **Start with the same exercise we did in secret #28, the "golfer kickbacks."** This simple move to help in the short term also helps rid you of pain in the long term.

   Do 3 sets of 10 to start. Over time, build up how many reps you can do to make your back really, really strong.

2. **For exercise two you are going to do hip drives against a wall.**

    You put one arm up on the wall lightly just for balance.

    You take the leg on the inside and you lift it up. Now let your hip drop casually and then drive it back until your leg touches the wall again. Then drop it out again, drive it up again and repeat.

    Do 10 to 15 or so reps if you can. Make sure they are really good contractions because you're teaching this muscle to get strong again.

    Do this 3, 4, 5 times a week, maybe every day if your back is hurting.

3. **The last exercise I recommend to get rid of back pain is the hip thrust.** It's an exercise invented by Bret Contreras to build your glutes without putting pressure on your back. It's also an exercise that's easy to recover from in the gym.

    Why hip thrusts?

    Another main cause of back pain is weak or imbalanced glutes.

    If your glutes aren't strong enough to do their job, your back takes over.

    Do bodyweight hip thrusts each time you do the other two exercises.

Do 3 sets of 10.

Build up the amount of reps you do over time.

Really squeeze your glutes each time you do a single leg or regular hip thrust.

The more you can feel your glutes activating, the more your glutes will start working for you on the golf course.

Secret Summary: It takes just 5 minutes a day to end most back pain for good using "golfers kickbacks," hip drives, and hip thrusts.

Secret #31 Never add weight to your swing in the gym

When I watch golfers on Instagram or Youtube, I'm surprised to see a lot of them making the same huge mistake.

They take their golf swing and add a resistance band to it.

Probably seems like a good idea for adding power and strength to your swing at first.

And I'm just as guilty as the next person for watching a pro pick up a weight plate and go through their swing motion with it.

But what it can screw with is how your brain has memorized and automatically performs your swing.

Think about it.

You spend thousands of hours training your swing to be just right.

You've made the tiniest tweaks to it to get it perfectly balanced, perfectly timed, and smooth.

Suddenly, you add weight to it.

This can change the entire sequence of your perfectly timed, perfectly balanced swing and send your brain mixed signals on how to perform your swing.

While you might end up with stronger muscles, the confusion between two similar but different moves ends up hurting your actual swing.

That's the last thing you want!

Secret Summary: Leave your hard earned golf swing alone in the gym. Instead, get stronger at basic full body movements like the deadlift: See secret #32 for more details.

Secret #32 Use movements that get you strong without messing with your swing

What kind of movements?

As golfers we need strong legs and powerful glutes and hips. We need mobility to make a full, smooth swing, and we need core stability to protect our backs.

For strength, the best thing we can use are big compound movements like squats, deadlifts, push press, and hip thrusts.

For power, we want to do explosive movements like medicine ball throws and sled pushes.

Core stability includes a lot of the exercise you see going around social media nowadays like the Pallof Press or one legged exercise with bands.

Mobility is getting the joints greased up and moving well with Jane Fonda type exercises like fire hydrants, hip raises, and chest openers.

When starting any new program, always start with 50% of the weight you think you can do to learn the motion of the movement correctly.

The reason is if you have an imbalance or a recurring injury, adding weight to an imbalance is the easiest way to turn it into a full blown injury.

To make things easy for you I've put together a full sample workout, mobility drills, warm-up and back exercises included.

Sample full body golf workout for beginners

Warm Up + Mobility

Bullet Proof Back Circuit

Single Leg Glute Bridge Hold - 2 sets of 20 - 30 seconds, rotate legs continuously

"Golfers Kickbacks" backs 2 sets of 10

Power

Med Ball Push Press and Drop 3 sets of 10 rest 30-60 seconds

Strength

Front or Back Squat (3 sets): 10 reps; rest 60-90 seconds

Dumbbell Incline Chest Press: (3 sets): 10 reps; rest 90 - 120 seconds

Romanian Deadlift (3 sets): 10 reps; rest 90 - 120 seconds

Single Arm Dumbbell Row (3 sets): 10 reps each side; rest 60-90 seconds

Glute Bridge (3 sets): 10 reps each side; rest 60-90 seconds

Stability

Plank (3 sets): 30 - 60 seconds; rest 30 seconds

Pallof Press (3 sets): 10 reps each side; rest 30 seconds

Secret Summary: Skip the fancy stuff. Do a little mobility, stability, and big compound movement work like deadlift and squats to become a powerhouse on the course.

Secret #33 Do two to three, 60-minute, full body workouts per week for maximum gains in minimum time

Most guys at the gym train a bodypart once per week, hitting chest & tris one day, back and bis the next, legs another.

Those big volume workouts are absolutely brutal.

I've seen guys that could barely lift their arms because they worked out so long and hard in one session.

Want to know what's ironic?

New research is showing it's also the worst way to workout for gains.

The reason is, your body can only handle a certain amount of work per week.

That's a finite number of reps and sets for a given muscle.

Do anything over that and your body won't get any benefit.

What's even more important to know is, your body can only handle a certain amount of work in one day!

Once they hit that "fatigue point," the rest of your effort is wasted.

For example, with glutes, one of the most important muscles for golfers, Bret Contreras, the inventor of hip thrusts, found through research that we can handle about 36 sets of total glute exercises a week.

If you were to do all the 36 sets in one day, a lot of those exercises would be wasted because your glutes would hit their "fatigue point" before you finished all those exercises.

A better way to do things is break those workouts into two days a week to get more of the benefits.

Break those workouts into three days and now you're stimulating your muscles more often while also doing less volume per workout.

The result?

Maximum gains in minimum time.

Secret Summary: Get in the gym! You will get 80% of the gains of even the most advanced lifters by lifting three, full body days per week.

Secret #34 Skip icing & cryotherapy get a massage instead

Want to know the fastest way to recover from a tough workout or an injury?

Cryotherapy and cold plunging for recovery used to be the hottest trends around.

But are they the best?

Turns out, icing, which can give you great mental benefits from dopamine release, offers nothing more than pain relief when it comes to recovery.As the Washington Post wrote…

Icing, it turns out, is like flossing: an ingrained practice that seems practical but is not strongly supported by clinical evidence. The oldest justifications for icing, dating to the 1970s, have melted under scientific scrutiny, some cryotherapy researchers say, and most scientific studies on icing haven't provided the solid results that would justify its popularity. This is true, they say, both for icing for daily recovery and for an injury.

Even the inventor of the RICE method no longer promotes it. "It's perfectly fine to ice if you want, but realize it's delaying healing," Gabe Mirkin said, "It's not going to change anything in the long term."

It's not that ice doesn't work, it's great for numbing pain, but science is showing it won't speed up your healing or get you back on the course faster.

Instead, the best thing to speed up recovery for sore muscles or heal an injury is another light workout. That's because getting blood flow to an area is the best way to help it recover.

A close second? Massage.

Why?

While there is some research on massages' ability to increase healing, what makes a massage really helpful is that it feels good.

Basically, it helps you relax, and check in with your body and how you're feeling during a little downtime.

And heaven knows we golfers need that.

Secret Summary: Icing is out. Massages are in.

Part 3: Drills

While this is a book strictly focused on little known golf secrets, I first built my community by sharing drills on Instagram.

I decided I couldn't put a book together without sharing at least 10 of my favorites.

So that's what I did.

I've added a handful of "Must Share" drills.

These drills still meet the criteria for "Million Dollar Golf Tips" - the 20% of tips that get you 80% of the improvement.

They take just a few minutes and many can be done in the comfort of your own home.

Even better, some of them include shoutouts to my favorite content creators, so you can get more drills like these from some pretty incredible golfers.

Again, if you haven't yet, go to **"Jasmincull.com/bonus"** to access your free bonus video series and daily tips email.

The videos will help tremendously if you are a visual learner like me. And the daily email gets you everything I'm learning and sharing the day it happens.

SECRET #35 The game changing one arm "Little Kid Drill" that will make a dramatic difference in every part of your game

Have you ever watched kids play? Watch a kid swing.

Kids almost jump off the ground.

That's because for them, the club is so heavy and falling so fast, they spring up to keep balanced.

As an adult, it's different.

Because you're strong enough, you can muscle your way through your swing and still hit the ball far with bad mechanics.

What a lot of people tend to do is take the club back and think they need to control the club with their arms.

They hit the ball using their arms instead of rotating their body to hit it. This is what creates lag in golf.

Kids can't. They may start swinging poorly, but their body naturally learns how to hit the ball far with mechanics, not strength.

They don't think about it. Kids let the weight of the club fall and their body to do the rest of the work.

There's no arms in it.

It's perfect. That's how they control the club and how they generate speed.

Real power comes from being able to grip the ground with your legs, rotate your hips, and let your body explode upwards as the club falls down into position.

If you want to swing smoothly and with power, copy what kids are doing.

One handed club drills are perfect for this.

This is one of those game changing exercises that can help your entire game, not just your driving and chipping.

The drill is pretty straightforward and simple.

You hit the ball with one arm only.

First, you're going to hit a ball with just your right arm only. What this does is takes your strength away. You're going to be surprised at how much better your mechanics are.

You'll also see what your real swing looks like when you don't have your second arm making adjustments.

Second, hit balls with just your left arm. The goal is to use your hips to rotate and let the club drop instead of driving through with your arms.

It might take a few swings to really get the hang of it.

As the club drops down into the ball your body uncoils in the opposite direction.

This is your body resisting the force of the club. It's like jumping off the ground.

As you feel your body pushing up, the club will actually accelerate.

That's exactly the feeling we want. For your body to go up instead of forward with the ball.

If you have a force moving down and you don't resist it, your body will go with it.

You do the exact same thing with your driver.

Let the club drop straight down to the ball, as you uncoil your body in the opposite direction.

The motion is the same for putting.

Use the weight of the club to hit the ball. Let the club flow. Keep your wrist passive and let your body rock back and forth.

There is no point buying expensive putters if you don't let the mass and the balance of them work.

While the one arm drills may seem simple and unnecessary, they help us hit the ball without muscling through it.

Using one arm helps train us to uncoil into the ball, hitting it smooth and pure, using the force of our legs and body instead of our arms.

If you're struggling with rising up to resist the force of the club, try the "Young Mcilroy Drill".

It may be a simple drill, but gets you feeling that upward motion instantly.

Secret Summary: Try these one armed drills to take arm strength out of your swing and get the feel for the natural movement of the club.

Secret #36 Too tense? Try this "Anti Tension" winner

Quick side note to go with the "Little Kid Drill" I just went over with you.

Tension is a pretty big problem in most sports. Over gripping the racquet in tennis, pickleball, and handleball can lead to some nasty results.

It can be even worse in golf, where you only get a few swings each hole.

If you're full of tension there's a little trick you can do to lighten up and let the club do its work.

Try this:

Take your little fingers off the club and your index finger on your bottom hand, so you're holding the club gently with just those inner fingers.

Now let your club fall up and down.

Gripping the club like this basically makes the club very, very light, allowing it to just fall onto the ball.

Secret Summary: If you're gripping your club tight enough to choke a chicken, remove your little fingers from the club on your next swing.

Secret #37 Copy this "Young Mcilroy Drill" to add explosive power to your drives

Looking to increase your power?

Try this.

Watch a young Rory Mcilroy's swing.

Notice his legs almost look like scissors as they extend and rise up powerfully. Also watch how the middle of his body moves up.

The head stays back. The power is exploding from his glutes and hips.

That's what you want and here's how to copy it.

1. Engage your core
2. Put a finger on your belt or midsection, and
3. Rise up using the hips and legs

Remember, the head isn't moving up. It stays back. The work is done by the glutes and hips.

It's simple but a great way to get that middle moving for more power.

This is the perfect drill to do before the "Little Kid Drill" because it teaches you to lift up and resist the force of your club moving forward.

Secret Summary: To get more power in your swing, engage your core, put a finger on your belt or midsection, and rise up using your hips and legs.

SECRET #38 Super easy & cheap drill to fix hooking and slicing

This drill makes me laugh everytime I do it because it reminds me of the video Rick Shield's made where he hit a box out into oblivion from what looked like the second floor of a Top Golf.

You don't need to spend money buying props for this drill.

Use your driver headcover, a towel, use any square box from around the house, or use a leftover piece of styrofoam.

As long as it's light and can make a line of some sort, it all works the same and can be a really useful training aid to get rid of slices and hooks.

Lay your prop on the ground.

If you're hitting slices, tilt your prop slightly to the right and hit the ball inside it.

If you're hooking the ball, reverse the drill.

Slant to the left and hit the ball on the outside of your prop to cancel out that nasty hook.

If you don't do it correctly, you'll hit your prop.

It's a great, instant feedback tool to correct your swing and start hitting more pure, straight balls.

Secret Summary: Use this drill and your headcover or a box at the range to stop hooking and slicing.

Secret #39 The "4 Tee" drill to strike the center of the ball and hit straight every time you putt

Have you ever wondered how professionals like Jordan Spieth can drain putt after putt with such consistency it looks almost magical?

That's what happens when you've trained yourself to start your putt on the line.

I like the "4 Tee" drill to train this because it's easy and a lot of fun.

You'll need 4 tees and a line tool.

Find your line and lay down chalk along the line.

Then, set up your tees along the line.

Put the first two tees down outside the middle of the start of your line, slightly wider than the size of the putter.

Then, twelve inches in front of that you put down two more tees. These go about a half a finger outside of the width of the ball.

The goal here is to make sure the ball starts on a straight line.

If you push your putter or swing slightly to the left or right, you're not going to get the ball through the tee.

Try this drill from multiple distances on the green and see how many times you can get the ball through the gates.

Secret Summary: Train yourself to putt straight on any line using the "4 Tee" drill.

Secret #40 The "Belt Buckle" drill for all the shankers, early extenders, and pullers out there

I heard an amazing story a few years ago about a woman named Grace Groner who took 3 shares of stock she bought for $180 and turned it into $7 million through the decades.

The moral of her story is that a simple plan followed for a long time will always beat a complicated plan that changes every step of the way.

That's what I like about the "Belt Buckle" drill I learned from golf pro Eric Cogorno.

He's got some great drills you should check out on his Instagram. You can follow him there **@ericcogorno**.

The "Belt Buckle" drill is the easiest way I've seen to "fix" early extension.

I say fix because we want to keep the extension, we just want it to happen LATER!.

Here's the drill:

Pick a target 10 to 20 yards left of the pin.

Push your belt buckle there.

Easy pease!

As a side note, early extension almost always happens because your brain is trying to fix an earlier issue like face angle, club path, balance etc.

Just make sure you've got these parts of your swing nailed and then incorporate the "Belt Buckle" drill.

Secret Summary: To hit straight, pick a target 10 to 20 yards left of the pin and push your belt buckle there.

Secret #41 A quick trick to crush drives and get rotating

I've noticed it's sometimes really hard for golfers to move their arms in line with their hips.

Instead, they muscle the ball a little with their arms instead of rotating and that really steals yards (and consistency) from their drive.

If you're struggling to make the change yourself try this simple Josh Park drill: Instagram **@jparkgolf**.

One reason I like it is because you can practice this movement anywhere, even without equipment.

He calls it "Moving the Line."

If you're at home, you can get a feel for it right now.

Get in your stance and put your club in your right hand (left if you're left handed).

You're just going to use one hand for now.

Pull the club back to about hip height.

If you were to look at yourself from the side, your right arm, shirt line, and pant line would now all create one straight line.

To swing consistently, you have to move everything together to turn through your shot.

So that's what you're going to do.

Keep everything in line, and then move that line together as you turn through your shot.

If you're at the range, line up four balls.

Move the line and hit one ball after another to get a feel for moving all together.

Once you get a good feel for this drill, gently rest your lead hand on the club.

Feel your hand staying on the side of your body, and notice your whole body is now rotating through altogether.

Secret Summary: To get your arms out of your swing use a one handed swing. Line up your right arm, shirt line, and pant line. Then move them all together to hit the ball.

Secret #42 How to master the weight transfer with a Bosu ball

Golf doesn't require big, bulky muscles to hit the ball well. What it does require is a well timed weight transfer.

Think of it as pressure in your feet.

A big mistake golfers make is keeping pressure in their back foot.

This means golfers transfer their weight back, but not forward.

The result is lack of power, inconsistent shots, and poor ball striking.

Oops!

It's the forward shift and foot pressure that's the most important. That's where the clubhead speed and power is generated.

Do it correctly, and your body doesn't move much left to right.

If you're not grabbing into the ground with your front foot at the right moment in your swing, your contact will suffer.

Try this simple drill to cement weight transfer into your brain.

1. Grab a bosu ball and a bench or box of similar height
2. Put your back leg on the bench, front leg on the bosu ball
3. Get into your backswing, feeling about 75% of your weight in your back foot
4. As you rotate, push your front foot weight into the bosu ball

It's a really cool feeling pressing into the Bosu ball with that front foot because you get instant feedback.

It's a feeling you won't forget and has direct payoff out on the golf course.

Secret Summary: Stamp down on a Bosu ball in this drill to get a pretty impressive forward shift into your swing.

Secret #43 The beach ball drill every golfer needs in their wheelhouse

This is one of the favorite drills invented by the guys over at Claws & Effect Insta **@claws_effect**.

Their mission is to make golf instruction simple.

And they're doing a great job.

When asked over and over how do you start your backswing, they came up with this amazing beach ball drill to get the feeling right every time.

Instead of a beach ball, I use a range basket. The principle is the same.

Imagine you are standing in an ocean of water just above your knees.

You take a small beach ball, balloon, or the range bucket in your hands.

Get into your stance and imagine you are in the water up to your midthigh.

Push the ball down and away from your body.

Memorize this sensation.

This is what really starts your swing, not the rotation of your body.

Really simulate pushing those palms down and away from the body, lower than when you first started.

That's the feeling you are looking for to start your backswing.

Secret Summary: Pretend you are pushing a beach ball underwater to start your backswing.

Secret #44 Make your practice a game within a game

Anyone that watched Brooks Koepka collapse Sunday at this year's Masters knows how brutal golf can be mentally.

Golf is easy in the "consequence-free" environment of practice. However, on the golf course you are accountable for every shot.

The sudden gusts of wind, unfortunate bounces, and imperfections in the turf make the stakes even higher when it counts.

The key is to make your practice much harder than your play. I find playing games within games is the best way to do this.

I'm talking about pressure practice drills like Leap Frog and Suicide or betting games like 3 Putt Poker.

The more you can break down each part of golf into another more challenging game, the faster your game will improve.

Here are a few fun and really popular games within a game to try out.

Secret Summary: Make practice harder than play with pressure drills like Leap Frog, Suicide, or 3 Putt Poker.

Secret #45 LeapFrog drill

This is one of Jordan Spieth's favorites.

The game is pretty easy and you'll want to play it for no more than 10 or 15 minutes.

The goal is to hit one putt after another within 6 to 18 inches of each other.

If you're doing short putts of 5 to 10 feet, the goal would be to get them within 6 inches of each other.

If you're doing long putts of 40 feet, the goal would be 18 inches of each other.

That's the first part of the game.

The harder part is right as you hit the putt, you have to predict whether or not your shot is going to make it within the right amount of inches to your last putt.

If you predict wrong, or your putt doesn't make it, you get a point. If you predict failure, you get a half point. Play with a partner or try to beat your lowest score each time.

1. Pick the range of putt you want to work on for the day anywhere from 10 to 40 feet.
2. Putt a tee marker down where you want your first putt to go

3. As you putt, predict the outcome before the ball gets there
4. Regardless of the outcome, putt again
5. The lowest score after 10 to 15 feet of putting wins

Secret Summary: Try to predict what your putt is going to do before it happens as you hit one putt after another within 6 to 18 inches of each other.

Secret #46 Narrowing Fairway drill

This is a great drill used by David MacKenzie, a performance golf coach focusing on the mental game of golf to train his athletes.

It's called the Narrowing Fairway drill because the idea is to start with a 50 yard fairway at the driving range, narrow it down to 30 yards, and finally down to 10.

The goal is to hit 3 drives at each distance before narrowing the fairway and starting again.

Only move on if you successfully hit all 3 shots down the fairway.

Make sure to set up each shot just as you would while you are playing.

If you can do this, the course is going to seem like child's play by comparison.

Secret Summary: Train yourself to hit pure shots down even the tightest fairways. Start by hitting within a 50 yard fairway at the range. Hit 3 shots in a row within the range before moving on to 30 yards and all the way down to 10.

Secret #47 Golf Suicides

Have you ever felt your heart pounding as you stepped up to the tee to hit a drive?

Nerves and adrenaline can wreck your game when you least expect it.

Golf Suicides is a great drill to prepare you for this.

It goes like this.

Pick a spot 10 feet away from where you're going to tee off.

You're going to race to that spot and back to the start three times before taking your pre shot routine.

The key is to get composed and your breathing under control before you step up to hit your shot.

If you don't focus on your breathing and get your heart rate calmed down, you can completely blow the tee.

And you don't just have to use suicides (the name for running back and forth between a short distance for reps).

Try 50 air squats in a row or if you're truly brave, 15 burpees.

Secret Summary: Simulate tournament adrenaline by getting your heart pounding before you tee off. Use suicides, airsquats, or burpees then focus on your breathing and try and calm down before teeing off.

Secret #48 3 Putt Poker

This game will leave you laughing all the way home from the course.

The fun here is you have two sets of score cards while you play - your actual scorecard and then your 3 Putt Poker scorecard.

Before you start, each player drops $5 in the pot.

With this game, it doesn't matter how many strokes it takes you to get to the green.

If it takes you 2 and your friend 5, doesn't matter.

The putting game within a game doesn't start until the green.

Once you get there, here's how you score the game.

1 Putt - Card

2 Putt - Nothing

3 Putt - $1 in the pot and better luck next time

4 Putt - Gets "the chip"

Normally the loser of the hole, usually whoever has three putts, gets the chip. It passes each hole to the loser. Whoever ends up with a chip at the end puts an extra $5 in the pot at the end.

All the cards you get at the end of the game are your poker hand.

When you finish your round, sit down and tally up who owes what to the pot and divvy out the poker cards.

Whoever has the best hand of cards at the end of the game wins the pot.

Go try it out and let me know what you think.

Secret Summary: Putt for dough. Get your shot to the green as close to the pin as possible and then lay it up for the best chance of winning 3 Putt Poker

Secret #49 Giant dice golf

Why SO SERIOUS?? I threw this one in because it's time to lighten up out there on the golf course.

For this game you need one big dice.

It can be the size of those fluffy car ones hanging from the mirror or you can go all out and get a giant inflatable dice you can roll around on the golf course.

The rules?

Roll the dice before the start of each hole.

Whatever you roll, that's the amount of clubs you get to play the hole with.

I posted a video on Instagram a while back, attempting to play a hole just with my driver.

It was hilarious.

Nothing is more fun than watching your friend use their driver to play an entire hole after rolling a one.

While you're watching them, remember the feeling you get.

Bottle it. That happy-go-lucky feeling is the feeling that's going to have you playing your best golf ever.

Secret #50 How to get top of the line clubs for half what everyone else has to pay

If you're serious about playing golf, you need the right equipment.

But you don't have to pay anywhere close to what everyone else is playing.

I started playing golf with a $100 set of clubs I bought from Sport Chek.

That wasn't as a kid.

This was as an adult.

I pretty much played a round a year, maybe two with them until 2020.

That's when I decided to switch from playing professional indoor volleyball over to golf.

Monet was tight.

Every extra cent I could spare went to lessons and actually being out on the course.

So I had to get a little creative.

I've found if you're a little creative you can get outstanding clubs for a fraction of the price.

Take this Scotty Cameron Putter for example...

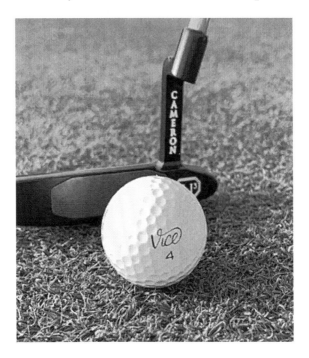

It's valued at over $800 USD.

But doing it my way cost just $410 USD.

Here's how I did it...

Instead of buying it outright, I found it on Facebook Marketplace for $300 CAD. That's around $230 USD right now.

I had Melvin over at Ironman Golf Refinishing Services do a Cerakote refinish, which normally costs around $250 CAD or $180 USD.

Melvin sent me a list of some of his most popular services to give you an idea of what refinishing costs.

He does satin metal finish and paint fills for $200, a Cerakote refinish like the one for my Scotty Cameron putter for $250, and a basic two-way face remilling for an additional $50. Any TIG welding to fill in dents is about $50, but the price varies. Laser engraving of image or text can also be done and again, the price varies.

You can find him on Instagram @theironman_golfrefinishing.

Another example is my new Callaway Paradym Triple Diamond driver I got for $400 USD also using Facebook Marketplace.

I took my original shaft off my TaylorMade driver and put a Callaway tip on it which cost me $50 down at the PGA superstore around the corner from my house.

I shortened my driver down to 44" and put a new grip on it.

All in all I was in for $470.

If I were to get that driver setup here in Canada, it would be $1200.

If you're like me and want to get some amazing clubs for a whole lot less than what everyone else has to pay, give Facebook Marketplace and refinishing a shot.

Secret Summary: It may take a little more leg work, but in the end, you'll have a beautiful piece of equipment for less than half what everyone else is paying.

Secret #51 The three tools every golfer needs to start dropping strokes immediately

#1 Camera Phone & Stand

I can't harp enough on how important videoing and video review are if you want to get better faster than everyone else.

Take videos any chance you get at the course.

To do that you need just two things:

1. a great phone camera, and
2. a solid stand to hold it

As for a great camera phone, I use my iPhone.

But you don't need an iPhone by any means.

Nowadays most camera phones are extremely high quality.

Android and Google also make great camera phones that compete in quality with the iPhone, like the Galaxy S23 Ultra and Google Pixel Phone.

When it comes to your stand however, you can't just use a normal camera stand. You'll need something that can stick in the ground without damaging the course.

I use the iRangeSports Stick EXT.

There's really nothing I've used that compares.

I first started using iRangeSports Sticks in 2021 and that's all I've used since.

What I like about the iRangeSports Sticks is it has a magnetic circle on the back my phone sticks to instantly.

The EXT model is adjustable to several feet in length, and it also fits in my bag like a golf club so it's easily accessible.

Not to mention, the metal spike on the bottom is thin enough to not damage the golf course, yet holds the stand still enough to get great footage of yourself golfing.

I talked to Gene at iRange to get a special deal for anyone that purchases my book.

Use code **JasminCull** at checkout to claim your savings on the purchase of your iRangeSports Stick.

#2 Alignment Stick

A lot of people when they're practicing are set up wrong with their feet.

They think they are aiming one way but their feet or body are aligned totally differently.

Many times they've been lining up wrong for so long, lining up the right way feels awkward.

That's where an alignment stick becomes game changing.

The alignment stick is key to teaching your body to feel how to line up correctly and visualize where to aim.

That's why every golfer needs to have one in their bag.

It's going to feel awkward at first for those that have been lining up wrong, until their body learns what it feels like to line up correctly.

Even worse, those people end up trying to adjust their golf swing thinking they are lined up right when really it's not their swing that's the problem.

If you don't have an alignment stick yet, make it the next thing you buy.

You don't need anything fancy.

For $5 you can buy a construction "reflective stick" at home depot instead of spending a lot more for a "golf alignment stick."

It's the same thing as an alignment stick but a lot cheaper because construction workers use these for markers.

#3 Club Cleaner

In 2021 professional golfer Luke Bodgan quit his job, sold his house and moved down to the US to try and play full time.

One of the most valuable lessons he learned in his journey was the more he practiced like he played, the lower he shot on the course.

So he changed everything he could about practice to match live tournament play.

One of the tools he used to encourage that behavior was to clean his grooves.

He began cleaning his clubs in between each shot just like he would on the course.

Rather than walk back and forth between his cart, he'd unhook his brush and carry it in his pocket.

After a while it hit him, *why can't I just carry my brush in my pocket all the time?*

That's when he went to work designing the Pocket Brush, a tool he still carries with him everywhere.

Luke's story is a reminder that a simple groove cleaning tool can be so much more than a cleaning aid.

Each time he cleaned his grooves, he was training himself to play on the course just as he had in practice.

Think about Luke's philosophy in your own training. How could a groove cleaning tool make a difference in your own game?

I recommend having two brush cleaning tools - one for your pocket and one clipped onto your bag.

The two I use are the Pocket Brush and the Grooveit Brush when I train and play.

You may want to try a few brands to see what you like best.

What's great about having a portable brush like the **Pocket Brush** is just that - it's small enough to be with you at all times so you'll have the proper control with your irons and wedges.

The **Grooveit Brush** is super easy to use. I like that it has a magnetic latch I can pull off my bag and then put back on super easy.

It has a built in water squirter so I can squirt a few drops on my club and use my brush to clean it and towel it off really quick.

If you're looking for either a portable groove cleaner and one with water to get a better clean, I've negotiated a special deal on both of these products for anyone who buys my book.

For the Pocket Brush use code **JASGOLF** as checkout to claim your savings.

For the Grooveit Use code **JCGROOVE** at checkout to claim your savings.

Secret Summary: Before your next round, make sure your golf toolkit includes a good camera phone, camera stick, groove cleaner, and alignment stick.

Final Thoughts: How to make this year the best year golfing of your life

Ever wonder why sometimes you play the best game of your life when you least expect it?

Karl Morris wrote a beautiful piece on it in Today's Golfer I sum up here.

Golf is a magical game.

Most of the time we enjoy it. We're out with our friends having a good time. We're relaxed.

And we play beautifully.

Then, pressure rolls around. We become quieter, more intense. We focus inward, breathe out, and typically blow it.

Why?

The ability to focus is a precious commodity. While a round may take four hours, just 10% of a round is spent golfing. The other 90% is spent on something else. And this is where the magic of golf is.

The art of playing your best round lies in what Chessmaster Josh Waitzken, who the movie *Searching for Bobby Fischer* was based on, calls Spontaneous relaxation.

From his book *The Art of Learning* he writes:

The physiologists at LGE had discovered that in virtually every discipline, one of the most telling features of a dominant performer is the routine use of recovery periods.

Players who are able to relax in brief moments of inactivity are almost always the ones who end up coming through when the game is on the line... Remember Michael Jordan sitting on the bench, a towel on his shoulders, letting it all go for a two-minute break before coming back in the game?

Jordan was completely serene on the bench even though the Bulls desperately needed him on the court.

He had the fastest recovery time of any athlete I've ever seen.

Golf, more than any other sport, has long periods of relaxation built in between holes.

In my opinion, great, consistent golfers do 3 things on the course to spontaneously relax for the 90% of the time they aren't golfing.

If you've ever played an incredible round of golf and are looking for a way to replicate that day over and over and over, try the following three secrets.

Secret #52 Build a mental trigger

If you want to be a great golfer in the minimum amount of time, you need a *mental* trigger, something in your head they can use to quickly snap back into a calm state.

Josh Waitzken shows you how to work backward to create a trigger in his book *The Art of Learning*:

When in your life do you feel most relaxed? Is it taking a bath, jogging, swimming, listening to classical music, or singing in the shower?

According to Waitzkin, virtually all people have one or two activities that move them in this manner, but they usually dismiss them as "just taking a break."

If only they knew how incredibly valuable harnessing their "breaks" could be.

If you can create your own trigger to connect a pre-set routine to an activity where you feel most relaxed, you can use that trigger before ANY activity to trigger a similar state of mind.

Since you can't take a bath anywhere you go, the idea is to slowly develop the trigger in increments so that the same relaxed feeling stays despite making the trigger shorter and more practical than, say , taking a bath.

Then, gradually alter the routine so it still has the same effect on you but is both shorter and easier to implement "trigger."

The secret is to make the changes to your "trigger" slowly so there is more similarity than difference from the previous version of the routine. This way the body responds the same to the trigger even if the routine is slightly shorter.

How to do it:

1. Find an activity where you feel in a state of flow.
2. Create a routine to use before this flow state activity
3. Do the routine for 30 days
4. Condense the routine by gradually reduce the time spent on each activity
5. Use condensed trigger to get into that flow state before you play a round of golf

For example, if jogging is your flow state activity, here is an example routine you can follow to trigger that state of mind before golf.

Sample Routine:

- Eat a light consistent snack
- 15 minutes meditation

- 10 minutes stretching
- 10 minutes listening to some Bob Dylan
- Go for a jog

Once you're consistent at the routine, you condense it. Here is an example of a quickly condensed routine to get to an optimal state in just 3 minutes.

You can condense your routine less dramatically than this to fit whatever amount of time you have to be ready.

Give it a try:

Sample Condensed Routine Starting at Month 2

- Week 1
  - Eat a snack over the course of 5 to 7 min
  - 10 min meditation
  - 8 min stretching
  - 8 min Bob Dylan
  - Jog
- Week 2
  - Eat a snack over the course of 5 min
  - 5 min stretching
  - 5 min Bob Dylan
  - Jog
- Week 3
  - Eat a snack over the course of 3 min
  - 3 min stretching
  - 3 min Bob Dylan

- ○ Jog
- Week 4
  - ○ Eat a snack over the course of 1 min
  - ○ 1 min stretching
  - ○ 1 min Bob Dylan
  - ○ Jog

Secret Summary: Triggering the right state of mind before golfing is the single most important thing you can do to have your best year of golf!

Secret #53 Ration your effort

We have all stood there ready to tee off thinking "I'm going to birdie or par this hole."

But not only can we not control the outcome, it's one that is three or four shots away still. We need to keep our mind on the shot at hand, not a future score. Like Padraig Harrington said:

"You can't make birdies, you can only create conditions for them."

The key is to ration your energy.

Get out there and enjoy yourself every moment you are not executing. Laugh, chat, enjoy the time you're not playing.

While average golfers seem to think it's a right of passage to throw their club and stomp around after a botched hole, save your mental energy to perform better. Once you've finished a hole, it's over.

Secret Summary: When it's time, give your shot your full focus and attention. The better you get at switching between focusing and relaxing, the better you will play.

Which brings me to the third and final step.

Secret #54 Start each hole fresh

Know what happens when you blow a shot and can't stop thinking about it? You blow a few more.

That's why it's so important to tee off at each hole as though you were starting a brand new game.

But how do you do that?

Build a trigger around your pre shot routine!

So maybe you do your pre-shot routine at home followed by a shower...

Maybe your "flow state" comes from reading a book or hitting a ball against the wall.

Whatever it is, if you use it after your pre shot routine, you will have trained your brain to perform in its most relaxed state each and every hole you step up to.

Secret Summary: Tie your flow state trigger to your pre-shot routine to start playing, consistent, smooth rounds of golf.

Conclusion: Make your next round count

There's a saying I like: ***"When you say MANY things, you say NOTHING."***

The meaning of it is you can only focus on one thing at a time.

Try to do many things at once, and you end up accomplishing nothing.

I'm sure you've experienced this phenomenon when you've sent an email or a text with more than one item in it.

Oftentimes the first part of the email or text is answered and the rest is skipped.

That's because our mind is wired to focus on one thing at a time.

The more things we try to juggle in our mind, the more our mental energy becomes split and unfocused.

What does this have to do with golf?

In golf, more than anything, focusing on just one thing at a time will have huge payoffs.

Take this book for example.

Instead of trying to practice multiple ideas at once, pick just one tip from this book and start there.

Once you master it, move on.

Maybe that's diagnosing the flight path of your ball so you can instantly correct your swing.

Maybe that's trying one of the back pain techniques so you can finally play without worrying about pain.

Or maybe that's trying out random practice the next time you drill at the course. Can you imagine how much better you will be when you are learning 100% faster than everyone else?

Everything you've learned in this book is simple, easy to do, and better still, WORKS.

What it does not do though is work the same for every single person every single time.

Perhaps what you are doing now is working a little bit some of the time.

So please do not try any of this once and tell me it did not work.

Try it over and over again until it becomes natural.

Each small change in your game could translate into multiple strokes off at the course.

I can't wait to hear how you're doing a week from now, a month from now, and a year from now.

Let's get out there and play!

THANK YOU

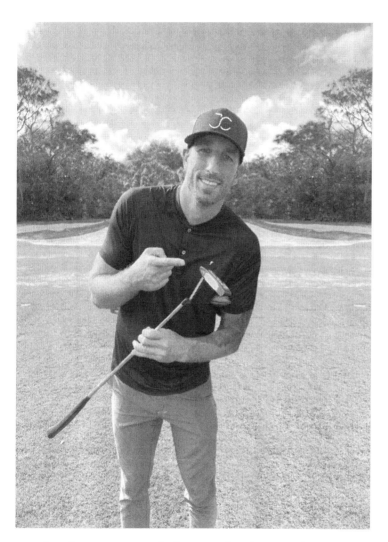

Thank you so much for purchasing my book.

You could have picked from dozens of other books but you took a chance and chose this one.

So THANK YOU.

I am truly grateful to you for getting this book and for making it all the way to the end.

That's why I'd like to ask a small favor of you.

Would you mind posting a review for me on Amazon?

It's one of the simplest ways to support small, independent authors like myself as I continue my crazy journey to the PGA.

And if you're on Instagram, message me @JasminCullGolf and let me know your story and how my book is helping you.

I can't wait to share your story with my readers.

To your best year yet,

Jasmin Cull

Follow my journey to the PGA on Instagram
@Jasmincullgolf

Printed in Great Britain
by Amazon

31703262R00090